I0480206

Memory Improvement

Complete Guide to Use Your Brain's Power, Learn Faster and Remember More

Jeffrey Turpen

Copyright © 2017 Jeffrey Turpen
All rights reserved.

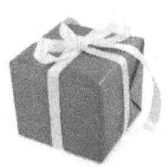

Your Gift!

We want to show our appreciation that you support our work, so we have put together a gift for you.

Just visit the link on the last page of this book to download it now.

We know you will love this gift.

Thanks!

Table of Content

Introduction

The brain is the most precious resource for a man, it is the center where we store memories, our experiences, where we handle all the functions of our body.

Learning to use the brain in the right way is vital to having a serene life and making the most of our potential.

Think for a second about your career, your study path, and your life in general. For a career you must always be responsive and able to remember every detail of each contract, if you are a student, you must bear in mind the concepts you study and be able to explain them with your words, and in everyday life, you must always be smart and able to avoid scams.

A brain active and able to function at 100% is your best ally in every challenge, and thanks to this book you will learn to harness its potential.

In the movie "Limitless" with Robert DeNiro and Bradley Cooper, the protagonist uses a drug to exploit 100% of his brain, but it's just a fiction, reality tells us we do not need drugs but only an efficient storage method, the right nutrition, and the right mindset.

The Latins had a very famous proverb, "mens sana in corpore sano" which means that the mind is healthy if the body is healthy. An active and healthy lifestyle is the fundamental principle of being healthy and having a brain that works.

Our brain is a muscle and requires training. If you want to become like Arnold Schwarzenegger you have to follow a hard diet, workout every day at the gym and have a determined mindset. Similarly to having a functioning brain, you will need to train it with specific workouts and proper nutrition.

In this book, you will discover all the best ways to improve your memory, to have a working and healthy brain.

You'll find all the best methods to have a photographic memory, to store concepts quickly and to study more in less time. You will know how to handle stress and fatigue and the best foods for your brain.

All the people who argue that memory training is unnecessary are liars, genetics may give us more talent than another person, but every person with training and commitment can achieve excellent results and have a brain worthy of Steve Jobs or Albert Einstein.

Let's start this journey in your brain with:

Memory Improvement: *Complete Guide to Using Your Brain's Power, Learn Faster and Remember More*

Chapter 1: How Memory Works

Before beginning to deepen Nutrition and storage techniques we need to understand how memory works. This study is long and complicated, and only the basic concepts will be expressed in this book.

Recent studies have shown that all the information we enter into our brain is stored in three different sections, where they are checked every time.

The first section is called "Sensitive Memory," retains the information sent by the sensory organs (nose, ears, eyes, fingers, tongue) but 75% of this information is immediately discarded. The remaining 25% is filtered, and only 1% is saved in the primary memory, the first layer of the brain.

The encephalon can abstract figurative impressions, verbalize what is learned and associate it with previous information. If multiple associations are possible, it is easier than what is learned to be remembered for longer times. Information is retained in primary memory for a variable period of seconds and minutes.

After this short time, some of this information is transmitted to the "Secondary Memory." But what decides what information can be sent?

The brain part that deals with this process are called Hippocampus.

The hippocampus is a nervous formation located on the lower edge of the lateral ventricles, above the cerebellum.

Hippocampus is part of the limbic system that is the brain area responsible for managing emotions.

In addition to the hippocampus, the limbic system belongs to the circumcision which covers it (para-hippocampal circumference), the circumference of the track above the so-called callous body and the broomstick.

All the components of the limbic system (closely linked to the hypothalamus) regulate the behavior of the primary needs for the survival of the individual and the species: eating, drinking, procuring food and sexual relations and, for an evolved species such as Man, the interpretations of signals from others and the environment.

This area of the brain deals with emotions, feelings, and therefore also our perception of reality.

People with mental problems often have difficulties with the Hippocampus and can not understand the reality around them.

We understand that Hippocampus is the brain window on reality, so it is strongly influenced by our emotions.

In a nutshell (we will deepen this concept later, it is a promise) if we associate positive emotions with a concept, it is much more likely that we will remember it easily. If a concept, situation, or whatever you want it causes a bad memory, then you immediately forget.

Think for example of the dentist and cake. The cake may be associated with a party, and if you walk past a bakery might think "wow, the cake of my birthday was delicious, it was made with cream and chocolate!"

A positive memory.

If we think of our dentist will remember "My tooth decay, it was painful, I will not go to the dentist, I'm afraid!"

A negative memory.

Often in psychiatric therapies, the most difficult challenge is to overcome the limitations of negative emotions and to remember negative experiences.

Personally, negative emotions and memories have to be recalled; they are life lessons that allow us to learn from mistakes and become more aware people. Hide evil and negative experiences is just counterproductive.

How is the information stored in the brain cell?

It has been found that if parts of the brain cell are destroyed by a stroke, no particular stored information is deleted. There are no areas where individual data is stored, such as on a hard disk of a computer.

Every information is broken down through an entire memory cell complex. If memory is recalled, it is sufficient to present a small part of the model (an association), and the whole model is rebuilt.

If different connections are used for similar patterns, you can create confusions and deja-vu.

The brain, in conclusion, it does not store the data as if they were a photograph, but through associations, with a procedure similar to the hologram, and it is possible, even when not all the data are retrieved, still obtain an entire image, even if it will be blurred.

In the temporary memory (short-term) occurs a rapid deterioration of the information, while the long-term memory stores information in a manner is substantially stable.

The information that arrives at Short Term Memory, if it is not subject to attention, starts immediately to erase even if, by repetition, it can be restored.

Short-term memory capacity is therefore limited: if the information is not repeated sufficiently frequently, it disappears. The compound of data present at the short time in the memory is called a repetition bearing. The information is stored in the bearing until it is transferred to long-term memory or until it is replaced by a new one.

Long-term memory is considered to be virtually limitless, but reactivating information can be prevented by the incompleteness of the associations required to identify it.

The immediate recall of information may be missing because it has not been transmitted to the long-term memory. The re-enactment of long-term memory information may be lost because there are not enough links to focus.

This theory also explains why some memories appear to be removed: such memories are inaccessible because their presence would be unacceptable to the subject because of anxiety or feelings of guilt that might trigger. They have not disappeared, but the subconscious avoids the significant associations being formed.

Individuals affected by amnesia do not forget everything, only personal items. This is often the case for an emotional trauma to which amnesia allows to escape. Often, part of those memories resurfaces when evoked by the right associations, many criminals often (as the Green River Killer) say they do not remember the details of their crimes, but in reality, they understood the seriousness of their actions and the negative feelings prevent them from remembering everything.

Chapter 2: The food for memory

Proper nutrition is the basis for a healthy lifestyle and to make the most of the benefits of a good workout.

Think of our body like the engine of a car. The engine is powered by gasoline, and if the fuel is of poor quality then sooner or later the engine will break. For our body the concept is the same, the food we eat is essential and eating harmful foods is counterproductive to our health.

Think of Arnold Schwarzenegger, do you think he has developed that physical only thanks to the gym?

No, the right combination was fitness and nutrition.

You will never get great benefits if you spend hours in the gym and then go to eat a Big Mac, and you will never have the body of a superstar if you eat correctly, but you train little or bad.

A proper balance of exercise and nutrition is the first step to train your memory.

Here are the foods that should always be on your table.

Fish

Spanish mackerel, anchovies, and sardines are among the most foods rich in Omega 3 fatty acids which perform a particular work on the central nervous system and development. They are crucial in childhood and adolescence because, in the development and learning phase, data is stored more easily in memory, making it work better.

So they should be present on a diet for the exams, and for all those who want to strengthen the mind.

Nuts

They contain many of the essential nutrients and are a great food for memory. In addition to a right amount of protein, they contain Omega 3 and Omega 6, Vitamin B6 and Vitamin E. In addition; nuts help regulate the serotonin level of the brain, a substance that controls appetite and mood.

Peanuts.

With properties not too dissimilar to nuts, peanuts are an excellent source of polyphenols and vitamin E.

Pumpkin seeds

Pumpkin seeds, often overlooked, are classified as food for memory because they are rich in vitamins A and E, Omega 3, Omega 6 and zinc.

Sunflower seeds

Particularly rich in vitamin E, but also Omega 3, Omega 6, vitamin B6 and minerals such as selenium, zinc, and magnesium, all of which have high antioxidant potential.

Wheat germs

It is an ideal food for memory, as it concentrates with antioxidants - such as Vitamins E and Vitamin B - but also mineral salts, essential fatty acids, and choline. To take advantage of its properties, it is important to eat integral grains. Grain buds, from the nutritional point of view, are also superior to the dried germ because the resources grow with germination. By placing grains in contact with water, a substantial enzymatic activity is created in the embryo, which significantly increases nutritional content.

Turmeric

This yellow spice - which we can find in curry, or use it individually to flavor the dishes - contains curcumin, an anti-inflammatory substance with beneficial action on the nervous system and in the prevention of Alzheimer's disease.

Spinach

This vegetable provides a mix of vitamins, including K and B9, antioxidants and mineral salts that protect the brain from aging.

Cabbages and broccoli

They contain vitamin C and folic acid (vitamin B9), essential to support memory, concentration, and attention, reducing the risk of Alzheimer's and other types of dementia.

Tomatoes

They provide lycopene, a valuable antioxidant that optimizes brain functions and protects against tumors. In this case, the cooking is very active because they release the lycopene, making it readily absorbable from the digestive tract. Blueberries.

Bitter enemies of free radicals contain even more potent antioxidant vitamins E and C, which help the memory and brain health. Blueberries also have anti-inflammatory properties.

Green tea

Besides being rich in polyphenols - very useful to fight cellular aging and decay of degenerative processes, thus preventing neurodegenerative diseases - brings caffeine, which as we have seen can have positive revitalizing effects on the brain and memory.

Coffee

Useful for caffeine content, although moderation is required to avoid the adverse effects of the substance, including inhibition of choline. When combined with dark chocolate, it is a great mix of food for the memory.

Dark chocolate

Cocoa is one of the best sources of flavonoids, which promote proper brain function, cognition and mnemonics.

Eggs

They are an excellent source of choline, one of the most important substances for memory. Even better then, eat eggs with moderation, to avoid the risk of ingesting too high amounts of fat and cholesterol.

Cod

Speaking of food and memory, it is among the most favorite foods to take choline and Omega 3.

As you can see are all pure and natural foods, no recipe too refined or rare foods.

This means that all so-called "miraculous supplements" that can develop your brain and increase concentration are just scams, a placebo effect at best or harmful medicines.

In nature, there is all the food we need to help our brains, avoid drugs and supplements, and eat more dark chocolate, green tea, and fish.

These foods should be taken in moderation, especially eggs, following a balanced diet and an active lifestyle.

Obviously, these are just tips, consider what foods you can eat (for allergies) and consult a doctor or nutritionist before beginning any diet.

Chapter 3: How to handle stress and fatigue

Proper nutrition alone is not enough to make the most of our brain; many external factors often prevent us from using our cognitive abilities to the maximum of their potential, they are called stress and fatigue.

The stress caused by work, by personal concerns, anxiety or other causes is one of the leading causes of amnesia. The brain can not handle all these stimuli and "switch off" all the memories that could increase stress.

A kind of protection (we have talked about it before, the Hippocampus is influenced by feelings) that "hides" memories that could fill us with stress and cause discomfort.

Stress, for example, is the reason for a problem called "dissociative amnesia," which is mainly affecting parents. These people leave their children (up to 2/3 years of age) in the cars closed under the sun for hours, with the result of giving these kids a horrible death.

Parents are convinced that they have left the children in kindergarten and continued their day. Only when they discover the baby's corpse, they notice their mistake.

Stress has caused this "dissociative amnesia" which means that the brain has "isolated" the cause of stress (in this case the child) and behaves as if it did not exist or as if the task had already been accomplished.

This is just one of the possible dangers that stress can cause to our mind.

Fatigue, on the other hand, is an enemy of study and memory because it prevents us from focusing in the best way and turns each study session into a marathon of effort. In a short time, we are tired; we can not concentrate and remember all the concepts we've learned.

It's better to clarify a concept.

The study should not be a "tour de force," a physical and mental challenge based on resistance, but it must first be a pleasure, and then a duty. Always try to avoid the exhausting marathon of study because you will not learn anything, in fact, you will get the opposite effect, you will be tired, and you will forget things much more quickly

The cliché of the student who is studying all night long for the exam is harmful, and it is the worst way to study.

So it is evident that it is essential to learn how to handle stress and fatigue in the best possible way.

And here's the first technique, the clockwork tomato!

What is the clockwork tomato?

Before explaining it, it is better to spend some words to introduce the concept of "procrastination."

Procrastination is a disorder/attitude that is not from memory, but the approach to every activity. The person who is procrastination always tries to delay anything, studying, write a business report, or start training at the gym.

In our case, it is useless to learn the techniques of memory if you are procrastinators. To fight this disorder you can read many great e-books and online courses, or ask for help from a doctor, but in this case, the tomato clockwork was invented.

Do not you think that you are a procrastinator?

The breaks in the study are necessary? Very true, but read this, and I bet that someone will recognize himself in this situation. You wake up with the idea to dedicate a whole day to study, then open Facebook to follow the dank memes, open YouTube to see if there are new videos, a ride on Instagram to see the photos of girls and is already midday, it is time to eat and then will you study later. 2 PM arrive, and you will go to bed, fall asleep and you will wake up more tired than before, but they are still 16, and so there is still time to study. So why not take another ride on the web? Then watch the clock, it's 20 o'clock, it's dinner time, and it's too late to study, and anyway today you've already done a lot of stuff (you waste a lot of time), so you can go out for the evening.

I bet this situation is familiar to many of you, and these people will only study the day before the exam, praying for fortune and meeting a non-strict professor.

This situation is the perfect portrait of a procrastinator, a person who wants to do so many things but can not get started, distracted easily and eventually lost time in useless activities.

To face this problem, and to help people who do not procrastinate to study better, the Clockwork Tomato was invented.

This method was developed in the 80s by Francesco Cirillo and has the ultimate goal of increasing the productivity of the individual, and its best field of application is certainly that of the study and can also be used in other areas.

The operation is effortless, use a common kitchen timer to ensure maximum concentration.

How?

All this is done simply by starting the timer, setting a duration of twenty-five minutes. The choice is not random, in fact, according to the author this is the time frame when the brain is at the maximum potential of its performance, and once this interval is over, it is necessary to allow a five-minute break to restore efficiency.

Whenever the break ends, you will have completed a "tomato," and the goal is to accumulate it as much as possible throughout the day.

Many people have received significant benefits in applying this technique because it gives you the incentive to concentrate you at your best. The constant ticking, at first, is annoying, but it will soon become a sort of mental trigger associated with productivity and work, so distracting will be more and more difficult.

A point of controversy is the 25 minutes of every single Tomato, many students found it a bit too short and requires too many breaks that, in a lot of cases, became counterproductive. So after some personal attempts, I found the perfect balance with 55 minutes of work and 5-10 minutes of pause. Keeping concentration for an hour should not be too difficult.

But subjectivity comes into play, however, personally making too many breaks means having too many moments when you are likely to close everything and stop working.

Before you have the best results, you must first test and evaluate in person what profile is best for each.

But always remember that the study should be pleasant and not a fatigue, you can stay in the 25 minutes of the first Tomato or increase up to 55 minutes as in my method, but always with no effort, otherwise the study will only be a waste of time and energies.

Chapter 4 - Memory Techniques - Part 1

Curse of the detective

The first method of memory is not a technique, it is a straightforward solution, but it can lead to great results. This method (or solution) is simple, so simple that many people underestimate and end up forgetting its beneficial effects.

It is a mutation of the so-called "Curse of the detective" (Readers who have seen "True Detective" may have already figured out).

Here is the explanation for those who have not seen the show or do not remember.

This is a typical problem for many detectives; they are investigating a case, collecting clues, controlling suspects, but failing to make any progress. They are not able to find the culprit and eventually the case is left unresolved.

But the solution is in front of the detective, is right in front of his nose, but he can not find it, and when he sees it is too late, and some innocent died.

Surely this is a melodramatic comparison, but it was the first association of ideas that came to mind thinking about the simplicity of this method.

This approach involves (indirectly) the Hippocampus.

In a previous step in the e-book, we said that the Hippocampus is influenced by our emotions and that all pleasant memories have a lot more chance of being memorized.

This concept is fundamental, and this method takes advantage of it in the best possible way.

In summary, it is necessary to create a pleasant learning environment, to stimulate the hippocampus to record all the information that we study, or at least the most.

First, listen to excellent music. The music does not have to be segmental or melodic, but it is vital that it is pleasant for you. Many people can study and memorize concepts while listening to "Sweet Child O'Mine" by Guns N Roses or the latest dance hits of the disco, while personally, I love the songs of Pink Floyd.

The important thing is that you like that kind of music because it will put you in a good mood and you'll be much more likely to remember what you read or hear.

You also need to find a way to make learning enjoyable. The real challenge is to make the lesson enjoyable.

In the comic movie "Road Trip" the protagonist is forced to study for a philosophical examination in less than 12 hours and is desperate. But his friend has the solution.

"I can teach Japanese to a monkey in 12 hours. The key is to make learning exciting."

"And how could you make the philosophy interesting?"

"Tell me your passion.'

"I love wrestling."

"Good. That's how I can make the lesson interesting. Socrates was the Vince McMahon of philosophy, was the forerunner, he has coached all philosophers."

"Go on."

At the end of the movie, the protagonist gets the most votes. Obviously, it's a movie, but the basic concept is correct. If you can find a system to turn a boring lesson into an interesting topic, you will learn it quickly.

But how can you make an argument appealing?

For example, are you a fan of fantasy?

If you are studying a history lesson, you can imagine the protagonists immersed in the fantasy world and think about their actions in that context or positive associate memories with an aspect of the lesson.

When I was studying electronics, I combined the design of the amplifiers to the disco music, and I was able to study better because I was thinking of pleasant memories of afternoons in clubs with friends listening to music. When I studied literature, I imagined the characters of the books in other adventures or made little comics with the scenes I read.

Creativity is a great ally in learning if used in the right way.

Chapter 5 - Memory Techniques - Part 2

Take Notes - The Cornell Method

The clipboard is a fundamental basis for every student, thanks to them you can study, review the lesson and try to understand what has been explained in class.

Taking notes is an art that is often overlooked by many people. "Ah, but what does it take to write something on a sheet? Just follow the speech. "

Well, I'm sorry to disappoint these people, but obviously it's not that easy to take notes for a long series of reasons, including time (you should be able to follow the lesson, understand the concepts and mark them practically at the same time), the understanding of what is being said and try to write in an understandable calligraphy.

In short, the notes require a particular method to be useful in the study.

The best method currently used by all students is the Cornell method.

This is (in very few words) a method of gathering the various data created by Walter Pauk in 1989, a professor at the University of Conell.

This method relates to the organization of the sheet to enter data rationally, allowing you to have a faster and above all effective consultation.

You can use an ordinary sheet of paper, or the so-called "Cornell Sheet" which is the "official" document of this method, ready to use for all students.

These forms can be downloaded easily from the Internet, but it is possible to use just ordinary sheets of paper, it is important to divide them into different columns correctly.

Quick advice if you use a regular paper sheet. You could write a lot of notes, so try to bring along sheets of appropriate size. As you know if you've been taking notes of any kind, the key word is only one, synthesis. You are not typewriters, and you do not have to do a complete transcript of all that is said in a lesson because at least 60% is just a useless attempt to stretch the broth.

The concepts should be short, use this mantra while you take notes:

"Short, shorter, even shorter."

If you look at the "Cornell" sheet, you will notice that the area is divided into three sectors, A, B, and C.

Notebooks should be inserted in the C sector according to the synthesis criteria.

Just enter the main topic of the lesson to the left, and enter the information that may be relevant or necessary, examples and everything you find necessary.

Do not write everything, but what you feel necessary. Separate each main topic of lessons or try to make connections. The argument should be on the left and all the details on the right.

In column A you have to prepare an index based on the contents of your notes, with the concept, keywords, important details of the sentences that sum it up. In a perfect job, you should be able to understand the contents of the articles just by looking at column A.

In the B column instead, you need to write a summary of the content of the lesson and any questions/insights / topics to be studied. Paradoxically, the contents of section C (the notes) are the least relevant on the page.

This method needs time to be exploited the best way, but once learned the mechanism it would be impossible to study without, thanks to its organization, which saves time and achieves outstanding results.

Thanks to this method you will be able to write notes very quickly and learn concepts in less time, and your memory will become stronger.

Chapter 6 - Memory Techniques - Part 3

The importance of conceptual maps

There are a lot of systems for taking notes and organizing all the information that was collected during the study. In the previous chapter, we saw the Cornell method for writing precise, easy-to-read, and most useful, notes.

Now we will talk about conceptual maps, a handy tool for every student.

Let's start from the foundation, what are the concept maps? This is a graphic representation of the concept we want to study. Visual representation should be schematic and reduced to the bone. A whole sentence may already be too much.

The significant advantage of conceptual maps is to make it possible to break a subject (even complex) into a series of small concepts (much easier to study) and to make connections of all kinds between different ideas, greatly simplifying the learning process.

A perfectly crafted concept map allows you to memorize each concept quickly and to explain it more simply. On the net, you can download already completed conceptual plans or install specific software to create the map that interests us.

But what is the procedure for creating a perfect conceptual map?

First, it is necessary to analyze the subject we want to study and identify the central concept, the one that holds the argument. This concept must be the center of the conceptual map, everything must start with him, and everything has to come back from him. Imagine the solar system, the sun is the concept, and the planets are the additional information.

Try to be very schematic as you make your conceptual map. The gift of synthesis is precious when it comes to studying and learning concepts. The more you manage to be short and the faster you will learn.

If there is a conceptual map, you can see colors and precise geometric shapes on the map. These are not random colors or shapes, but correct choices. Shapes and colors must indicate the degree of importance of concepts and their links. There is no universal system of colors and shapes; each person uses the colors and shapes that he or she wants.

To sum up, to create a concept map you must first identify the core idea and all the corollaries that you want to insert into the map, then you need to find the logical concepts that bind them (not to be forced, but natural), to develop their own colors and geometric shapes and then create the map.

So the concept maps are a valuable aid to study, in fact, help us to store all the concepts efficiently and to understand better what we are studying, are easy to make and can be found already compiled online. Each student can learn a concept map in seconds, and the teachers will encourage their use. Finding the geometric shapes and colors that you like is very simple and will allow you to customize your maps and make them even more unique.

Are not you still using it? What are you waiting for?

These two methods are indispensable for students and for those who want to memorize something quickly. Do not underestimate them because they may seem simple, and remember that simple things are always the most productive.

Chapter 7 - Memory Techniques - Part 4

Photographic memory

What is the photographic memory?

It is a hoax.

I'm sorry to destroy your expectations, but I want to be honest with you.

So when you see a show (such as "Suits") where the protagonist has a prodigious memory, remembers everything and can store a whole book in seconds, always bear in mind that it is fiction so what you see does not have a real counterpart.

Otherwise, we might think that the sound propagates in space because the Star Wars battles have a beautiful sound.

Therefore, "photographic memory" does not exist, but in nature, there is something similar, "eidetic memory."

What is "Eidetic Memory"?

It is the ability to recall the images with extreme precision, even after only a few seconds of exposure.

However, this mnemonic capacity lasts ten minutes, after that the mental images tend to fade. It is also present in only a small percentage of children (between 2% and 10%) and completely disappears in adulthood.

The fact that the photographic memory is a hoax does not mean there are not people be able to store, even in a short time, information seemingly impossible to remember. How do they succeed?

The alternatives are two:

They have a genetic predisposition

Or

They have learned to use to perfection some memorization techniques.

These techniques (just like those that have already been described) require a long time to be used to perfection, but here are some effective tips to increase the chances of developing Eidetic memory.

1 - Increase your knowledge of a single topic.

This trick will allow you to become experts in a field. Find a subject that interests you and continues to study it, you will always find new lessons to be played, new topics, and in a short time, you will become real experts in the industry.

For this reason, in one area, which is good it becomes more and more skilled. And who is poor is becoming increasingly scarce.

In the first case, new information increases the "global sense" of the previous ones.

In the second case, however, every new information increases confusion.

Studying the same topic every day you become the expert, because you'll know exactly what you were studying yesterday and your brain will automatically create connections between topics, accurate automatic concept maps.

2 – Draw

Drawing is a beautiful art, and some people are born with a talent that can make them unique, like Michelangelo, Leonardo Da Vinci, Picasso, Salvador Dali, Roberto Raviola (Magnus) and much more.

For our course, there is no need to be a painter or a talented artist, but drawing is very useful for developing eidetic memory.

The exercise you can perform is straightforward, look at a place, an object, a person, and try to draw it. In this way, your mind will remember many details more quickly and strengthen your memory.

If you are not artists (like me, the worst drawer in human history), you can describe the scene, object, or person by writing a description, even in this case, the brain will remember a lot of details and your eidetic memory will grow.

3- Use the infographics

Infographics are an interesting method of study, which allows you to use a chart to explain a concept. This method is very useful in economics, with a graph you can briefly account for a budget, company goals, profits, and losses.

Using an infographic to will strengthen your visual memory. The infographic is never boring, and our brain is particularly attracted to colors and shapes, making a comparison is a more "pleasing eye-view" of a conceptual map.

The brain will get many benefits from this infographic, whether you should just consulate it, or if you realize it. The creative effort and the use of images will help the development of eidetic memory.

In conclusion, the "photographic memory" that we see in many movies and books do not exist; it is a trick created by writers.

Some people have this incredible talent, but they are sporadic cases. However, there is a memory that can use images to store and instantly call up a series of memories, eidetic memory. These exercises will not turn you into a genius, but they will help your brain develop a new competence, thus expanding eidetic memory.

The important thing is the constant training; I wrote that the mind is a muscle, and as such must constantly be trained, otherwise it will never reach the physical form we want.

Chapter 8 - Memory Techniques - Part 5

How to read and memorize quickly

Most of the concepts we study and try to remember come from reading a book. For this reason, it is necessary to develop a system to read quickly and to learn a concept immediately. Many memory techniques can help us quickly store a book, what we will see now is called PhotoReading, and according to many scholars this method, if used well, allows to store 100 pages in 20 minutes.

But be careful: memorizing a concept does not mean to understand it. The study and understanding are needed, the worst possible thing is to recite a concept like a parrot, without understanding the meaning of words.

With this method, you will have more time for understanding, because the memorization stage will be fast and efficient.

STEP 1.

The first step to applying the PhotoReading system is to realize your goal, to become aware of what you are about to do.

It is therefore essential to empty your mind from any extra thought and to affirm your act of will: "I'm going to memorize a whole chapter."

It may seem like an unnecessary step, but it is not, is a way to prepare our minds to receive new information and to "unleash" our willpower. Initially, avoid unnecessary thoughts will take some time, but with a bit of workout, you will be spontaneous.

STEP 2. BROWSE QUICKLY THE CHAPTER.

Quickly scan the section you need to study. Pay close attention to paragraph titles, bold words, on any visual indicator.

An old military adage teaches that the time spent for reconnaissance is never wasted time!

This depends on the fact that through the preview of the materials to be studied, we allow our minds to begin cataloging information as if they were files to be filled.

More orderly will be the reconnaissance and more accurate and complete will be your mental archive.

In this step, it may be useful to prepare a quick conceptual map.

STEP 3: FAST READING TECHNIQUES.

The most difficult step in PhotoReading is the time when the brain absorbs information directly from the pages we are about to study.

To read, or to collect information from the book quickly, you can use the fast reading technique you prefer.

PhotoReading is based on a different way of "looking" the book. Not as a text to read every word, but only the information that interests us.

Many experts recommend beginners to associate with a fast reading technique, a preliminary phase in which a pencil is emphasized, the information that interests us.

My method has always been to highlight with a pencil the passage that interested me and just studying it. The time I spent on the study was minimal, it is said that "less is more," a compelling study, with a method studied and used with a proper method, can produce excellent results in a short time. Three other fast reading methods can be:

a) Use a pen, a pencil or your finger to scroll through the words quickly. Your eyes will get used to following the finger, reading much faster. However, this method requires a training period, especially to find the speed that suits you.

b) Try to read a whole sentence at a time, do not focus on a single word, slowing down the reading process enormously.

c) Look at the words you are reading quickly, this method is an evolution of the method 1, and allow the eye to scan a greater number of words.

Online you will find many free tools to work out these methods of fast reading.

STEP 4: ACTIVATION.

By reading fast, your mind will have absolutely no control over the information you have read.

This means that immediately after reading the book you will have the feeling of not knowing anything.

No problem, it's perfectly normal.

Thus, the fourth phase begins the activation. This involves recalling information that is unconsciously captured in mind, one of the most favorite memory recall techniques. Within a few weeks, your storage time will decrease by as much as 50%. Memory recall techniques are many and varied, here are some of the main ones:

1) Meditation. Concentrate, relax and meditate, listen to relaxing music, and let your mind recover all memories. You can use an App as Headspace to meditate in the right way.

2) Caffeine, coffee is a great ally of memory, a caffeine pill is one of the best solutions for recalling memory.

STEP 5: AUTOVALUTATION

The fifth step is optional. And it is recommended for students who have to face an oral question or exam. It consists in self-evaluation.

The best way to figure out whether or not you understand what you have studied is to put you in the shoes of the professor and ask questions.

Do it even after using the PhotoReading. PhotoReading is a complicated technique, but once learned it could really help you speed up your study and quickly remember what you read.

Do not be discouraged immediately; an efficient method always takes a long time to be used to perfection.

Only a fool would believe to achieve excellent results in a sector with little effort and in a short period of time.

Chapter 9 - General tips

We've studied some storage methods, but the list could be much longer, but these are the main ways, the most useful and straightforward to use.

Additionally, here are some helpful tips for integrating habits that can help us further improve our memory.

Tip # 1 - Meditation

Meditation is not a new-age fashion, but an effective way to get in touch with ourselves and expand our minds.

As already written, meditation is an excellent method for recovering memory and also completely delete the stress of our lives.

Integrate meditation into your lifestyle (it does not take too long, even 10 minutes are useful), you can use audio books, music or App as the Headspace mentioned above to meditate from your home.

The results will be amazing.

Tip # 2 - Sleep

Sleep is vital for our health. If we do not sleep enough, we will be tired, with no energy and we will not be able to memorize anything in the right way.

Once again, the study should not become a marathon. If you are forced to study on the last day, it means you are a procrastinator or your research method is ineffective. The only result you will get will be to waste time, waste energy and do not remember anything.

During the night, in fact, in our brain, there is some consolidation,

During the day we encounter many interferences that make us forget how much we learned but sleep returns to memory the notions and abilities that seemed to have been only partially erased.

A proper pace of sleep not only to remember but also to learn better: if we have slept enough, our brain is more alert, absorbs more information and holds it longer. Needless to squeeze our forces, investing in sleep is a great technique to deal with the day.

Tip # 3 - Physical Exercise

Physical activity is not only an excellent way to lose weight, to cure our body, and to eliminate stress, but it is also an effective system for improving memory.

In fact, during exercise, oxygen circulation in the blood is greater, and this is a very positive effect. The brain, therefore, will have the ability always to have new cells and a greater supply of oxygen.

Physical activity after the study allows you to memorize the concepts and understand them in less time.

My personal experience is that 10/15 minutes of jogging before writing allow me to be much more creative and full of energy. Yoga is also a great physical activity, especially the 5 Tibetan rites.

Tip #4 - Avoid distractions

Distractions are an enemy of the study. In this era of Smartphone, Facebook and Instant Messages this enemy is stronger than ever.

Think of the time spent on Facebook or watching videos of kittens on YouTube. Time wasted a perfect procrastination.

Do not get me wrong, distractions and breaks are needed (they are part of the Clockwork Tomato), but the pause must only be a break for a few minutes, it does not have to be an excuse to waste time.

Willpower is a great ally to fight distractions, but often alone is not enough, and then technology can help us with sites and applications that will allow you to obscure a site for a certain amount of time, such as Freedom.

This is not about censorship, but only to avoid distractions for a period of time, which must be only dedicated to the study.

Conclusion

The mind is powerful and is still partially unexplored. The memory techniques and personal development courses are regularly updated, and every day a student can develop a new rapid storage method.

These methods are theoretical, to put them into practice, you must first know your limitations. Each person has a different brain; some people can remember a name or face instantly, others can make math calculations in a second. The brain of each is different, and therefore it is necessary to find the most suitable method for each person.

Experiment each method to find the one that suits you and modify every suggestion according to your needs.

But above all, do not hope for quick results in a short time. Achieving successful outcome is the product of months of training and requires the utmost commitment and perseverance. Do not be frightened by the difficulties and in the end, the results will be excellent.

So use your mind and memorize the concepts, it is easy thanks to this guide :)

Your Gift!

We want to show our appreciation that you support our work, so we have put together a gift for you.

bit.ly/2u7pdNL

Just visit the link above to download it now.

We know you will love this gift.
Thanks!

www.ingramcontent.com/pod-product-compliance
Lightning Source LLC
Chambersburg PA
CBHW070929220526
45468CB00005B/1707